LITTLE BOOK OF

FIT AT FIFTY

LITTLE BOOK OF
FIT AT FIFTY

First published in the UK in 2013

© Demand Media Limited 2013

www.demand-media.co.uk

Printed and bound in Europe.

ISBN 978-1-782811-82-4

The views in this book are those of the author but they are general views only and readers are urged to consult the relevant and qualified specialist for individual advice in particular situations.

Demand Media Limited hereby exclude all liability to the extent permitted by law of any errors or omissions in this book and for any loss, damage or expense (whether direct or indirect) suffered by a third party relying on any information contained in this book.

All our best endeavours have been made to secure copyright clearance for every photograph used but in the event of any copyright owner being overlooked please address correspondence to Demand Media Limited, Waterside Chambers, Bridge Barn Lane, Woking, Surrey, GU21 6NL

In no way will Demand Media Limited or any persons associated with Demand Media be held responsible for any injuries or problems that may occur during the use of this book or the advise contained within. We recommend that you consult a doctor before embarking any exercise programme. This product is for informational purposes only and is not meant as medical advice. Performing exercise of all types can pose a risk, know your physical limits, we suggest you perform adequate warm up and cool downs before and after any exercise. If you experience any pain, discomfort, dizziness or become short of breath stop exercising immediately and consult your doctor

Contents

Foreword
by Diana Moran

Health Broadcaster
and Journalist

Learn to look after your health, because as the years go by good health will help you enjoy today's increase in longevity. The medical and physical benefits of keeping fit are improved circulation, digestion and a stronger heart. Exercise builds strong muscles and bones, increases your flexibility and co-ordination. Combined with a well balanced diet, exercise helps control weight and improves shape. By making the best of yourself you will experience a sense of well-being, feel relaxed and more confident in your life.

It's all common sense really – fitness is about being able to do the things you want to do. But being fit should be a necessity of life - not just an option! Your individual level of fitness will depend on your

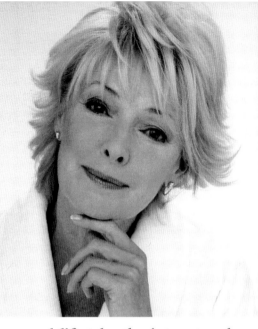

personal lifestyle, the interest and commitment you have to looking after your health. And the good news is that for those people who get it right, there may be a decrease of some physical ability in their 60s, others later, and some, not at all! Many individuals enter advanced old age still performing at the level of younger adults.

Just half an hour of moderate physical activity five times a week can help, and significantly improve your health and well-being. Fitness workouts, dancing, gardening and other sports which make you feel warm and slightly out of breath are most beneficial.

There may be some bodily changes with age, but good habits will benefit you as the years roll past. The Little Book of Fit at Fifty can help you maintain fitness. My programme Easy Fit, is also available on DVD to complement this volume. So take the time to make the effort, and enjoy many more years of active life.

"If you don't use it, you may lose it"... applies to both body and mind! At the ripe old age of 74 I should know!

Important

Not all exercises are suitable for everyone and this or any other exercise programme may result in injury.

Before starting any exercise programme you should consult with your doctor to reduce the risk of injury, especially if you suffer from heart disease, have high blood pressure, joint problems, back problems, are overweight, have an illness, injury or are convalescing.

The instructions and advice presented are in no way intended as a substitute for medical counselling. The creators and distributors of this book do not accept responsibility for accident or injury as a result of the exercises and advice therein.

As with any exercise programme you should start slowly and build up gradually. If a movement hurts – stop! Do what you can today and try again tomorrow. If pain persists – check with your doctor.

Check the location and surfaces before performing any exercises in your home.

Clear a space and check that surfaces are not wet or slippery. Ensure that any support and equipment you use is strong

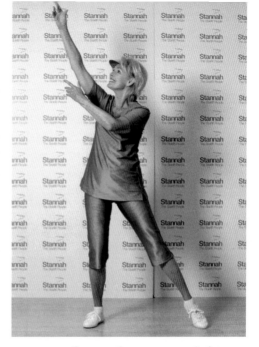

enough to take your weight.

Make sure you are warm enough and wear layered loose clothing that can be discarded as you warm up!

Don't exercise until at least an hour after meals and keep drinking water to avoid becoming dehydrated.

Chapter 1

Warm Up and Stretch

Stand with your feet just more than shoulder width apart and stretch right up to the ceiling with your arms and then push it away and repeat several times.

Step 1

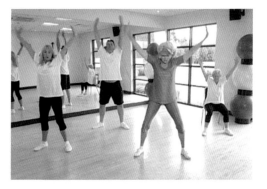

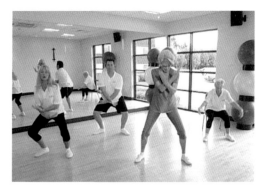

Step 2

Turn your head to the right, hold for a second, bring it back to centre and then turn it to the left. Do it again, but this time try and take the head a little further round on each side.

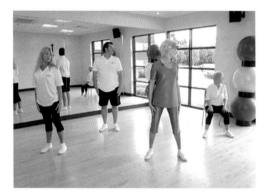

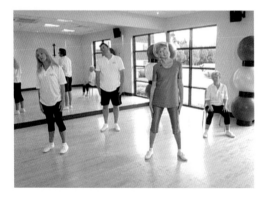

Take your ear to your shoulder, stretching out the side of the neck. Hold for several seconds, come back to centre and do the same on the other side. Repeat for a second time.

Lift one shoulder up towards your ear and then push down with your hand. Repeat the exercise on alternate sides several times.

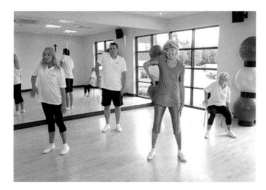

Step 1

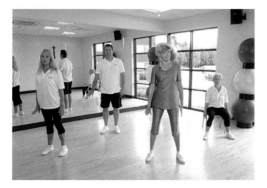

Step 2

Roll one shoulder backwards, pulling the shoulder blade back, and then the other one. Repeat the exercise on alternate sides several times.

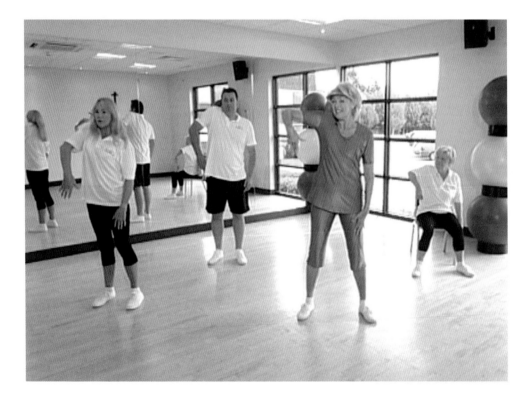

Push down to one side and then to the other. If you prefer you can also bend the knees. Repeat several times.

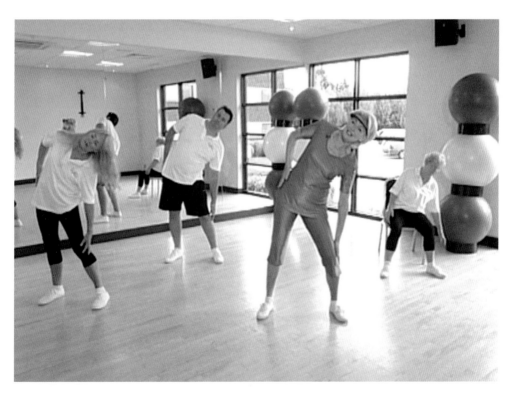

Put your hands out in front of you. Twist the upper body, but keeping the hips facing forwards at all times. Twist to the right, come back to the centre and then to the left, and back to the centre. Repeat several times.

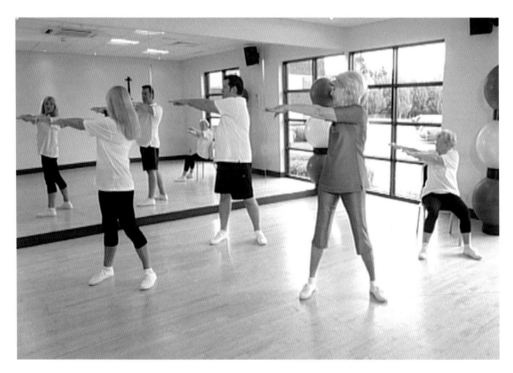

Put the right hand into the small of your back and either ease your arm or pull your arm back with the other hand to get a good stretch in the upper arm. Hold it for about 8 seconds and repeat on the other side.

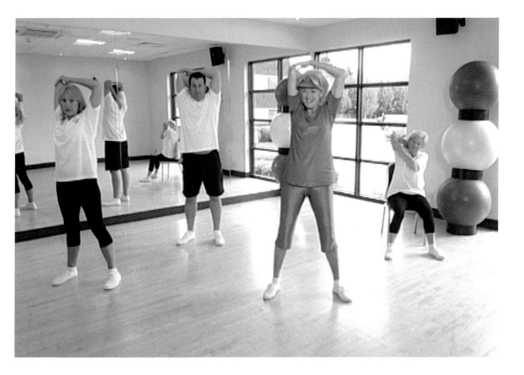

To stretch out your shoulders, put your hands in front of you and imagine that you are hugging a big beach ball. Pull in the tummy, slightly bend the knees, drop your head down between your arms and stretch out around your shoulders and back. Hold for about 8 seconds.

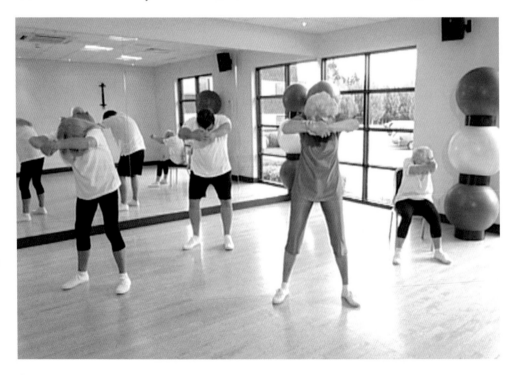

Take your hands behind you, grasp your hands, pull your shoulders back and then lift your arms up a little bit. Hold for 8 seconds.

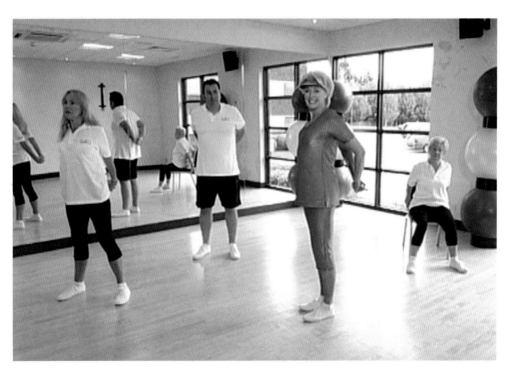

Stand with your feet just more than shoulder width apart, and transfer your weight from side to side, adding a little swing each side with your arms. This is perhaps best done in time to some music. The higher you swing your arms, the more aerobic you will get. Do this for about 30 seconds.

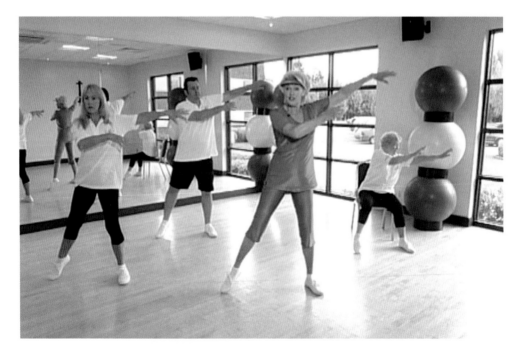

Take the right arm and shoot it like an arrow across to the opposite side, bending the knee, and then do the same with the left arm. Again, this is best done to the rhythm of music. Repeat several times.

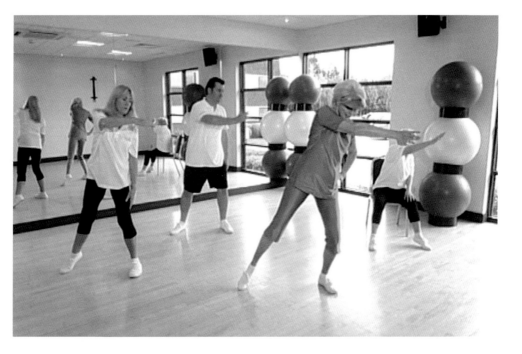

Continuing the above exercise but start to bend your knees a little more and take the exercise down as low as is comfortable for you. Maybe you can even touch the floor. Gradually come back up until you are doing the exercise standing upright again.

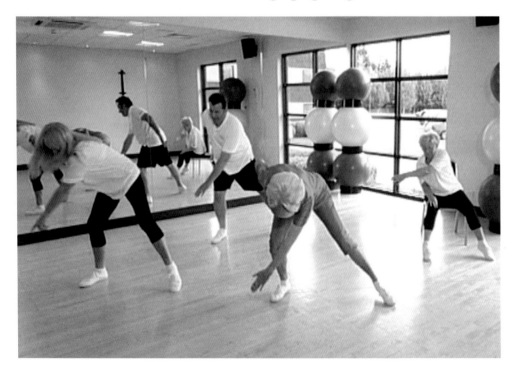

Continuing with the same movement, this time go up higher, really reaching up as much as you can every time. Repeat several times and then come back to doing the movement across the body again.

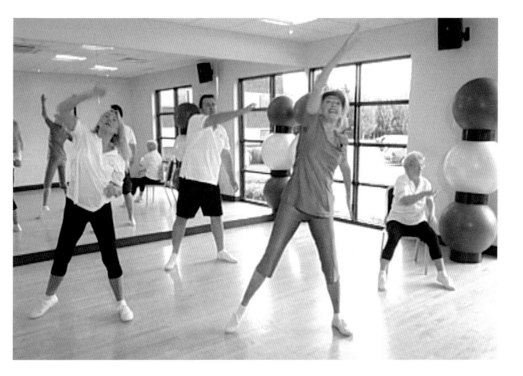

Stretch the right hand right up to the ceiling and take a deep breath. As you breath out, bend over to the left stretching out your side and hold for 8 seconds. Come back to centre and repeat on the other side.

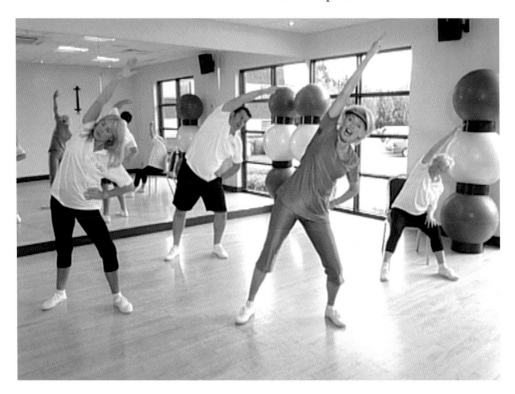

With knees slightly bent and with hips very relaxed, move your hips from side to side loosening the hip and lower back area. Continue the exercise for about 20 seconds.

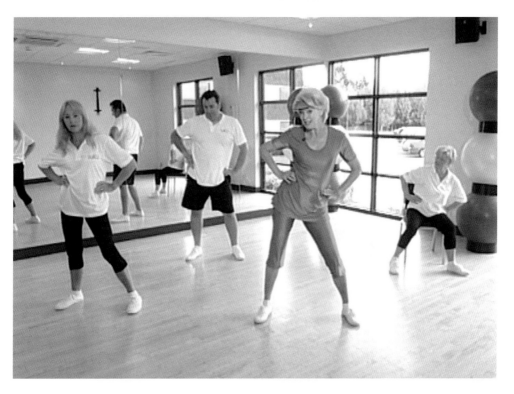

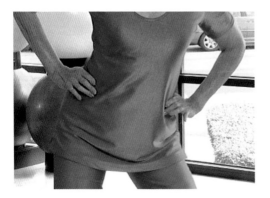

To loosen the hips even more, change the side-to-side movement into a circular motion and circle the hips round and round for about 20 seconds.

Standing with feet quite wide apart and with your knees in line, but not over your toes, simply sit down keeping the upper body upright stretching out the inside of your thighs.

Hold for about 30 seconds.

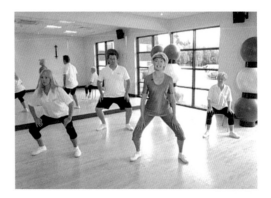

Add a neck stretch to this by dropping the head down and again hold for about 10 seconds.

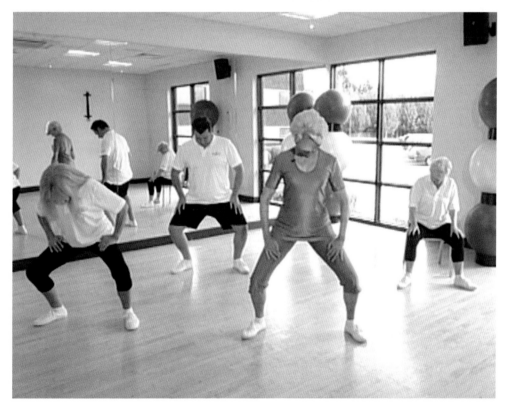

Stand with your feet together and hands on your hips. Stretch one leg out and place your heel on the floor in front of you, then bring it back and put your toe on the floor – heel and toe, heel and toe etc. Repeat on the same leg for about 20 seconds then do the same on the other leg.

Step 1

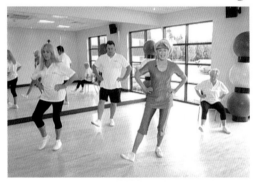

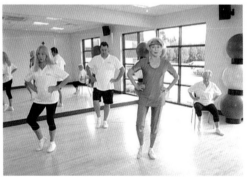

Step 2

Put your elbows closely into your waist and make fists with your hands. Repeat the last 'heel and toe' exercise but this time as your heel goes down your arms come up and as your toe touches the floor your arms come down working the biceps as well. Keep the arms tight into your side and the movement up and down only comes from the elbow. Repeat on one side for about 20 seconds then continue on the other side.

Step 1

Step 2

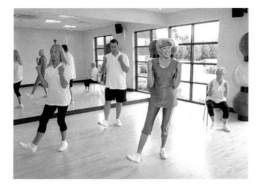

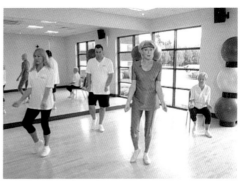

Repeat the 'heel and toe' exercise again, but this time working the wrists as well. With your elbows tucked into your side and palms of hands facing upwards to start with.

Step 1

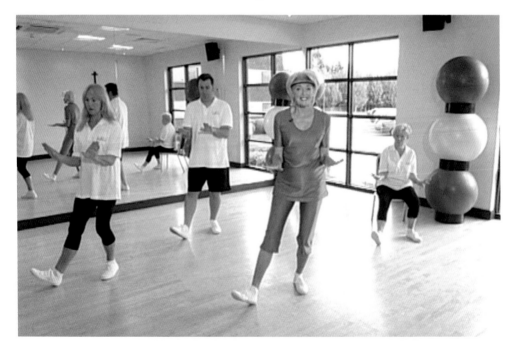

As you do your feet you need to turn your hands one way and then the other, twisting the wrists each time. Repeat for about 20 seconds and then continue with the other leg.

Step 2

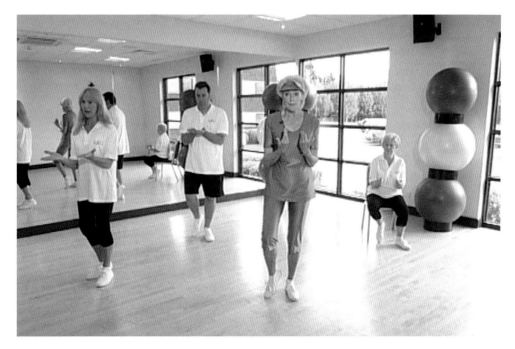

Stand and then take one leg back behind you and push the heel down and hold for 8 seconds. Come back to centre and with the same leg, bring it forward a little way. Bend slightly forward and lift up the bottom on the side where you're stretching. Hold for 8 seconds. Repeat on the other leg.

Step 1

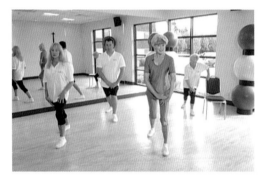

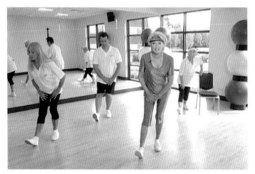

Step 2

Lift one leg and hold behind your bottom, keeping the front thighs parallel. Push your hips forward a little to increase the stretch. Hold for 8 seconds and repeat on the other leg.

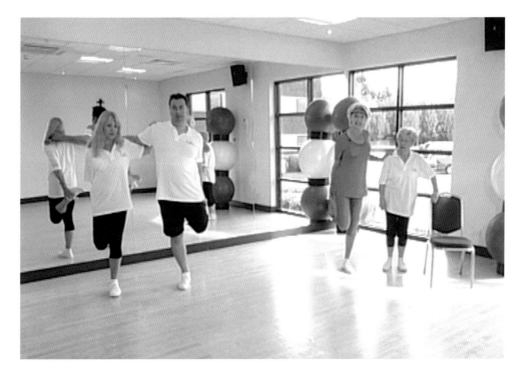

Chapter 2

Cardio Work

N.B. These exercises are easier and more fun to do in time with some music. If you want to flow seamlessly from one exercise to the next, then just repeat the first explained 'Holding Pattern' routine in between each different exercise.

Holding Pattern: March on the spot for 8 beats, then move forward on the next 1, 2, 3, 4 and march on the spot – 1, 2, 3, 4, then back 1, 2, 3, 4 and march on the spot 1, 2, 3, 4, 5, 6, 7, 8. Pump the arms throughout. Repeat this sequence.

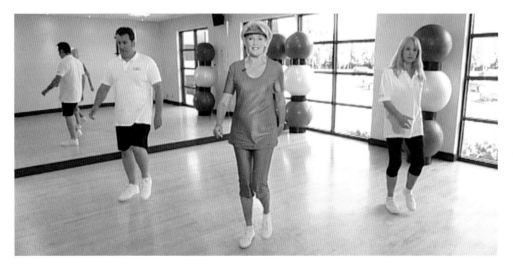

Keeping in time with the music, with one leg moving on every beat, move one leg forward and slightly to the side and then the other leg forward and slightly to the side (like a 'V' shape) then on the next beat

Step 1

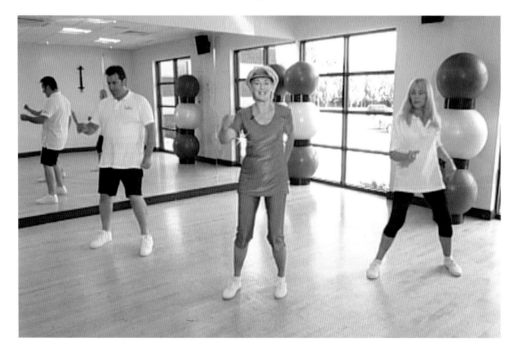

move the first leg back and then the other leg back in time to the music. You can also add some 'roly poly' arms to this exercise if you wish. Keep doing this for about 30 seconds.

Step 2

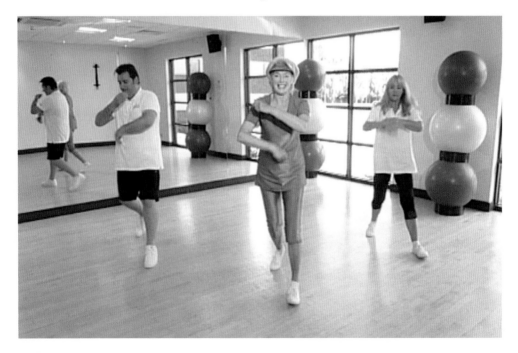

Step forward with one leg and as the other leg comes forward to join it, lift it into the air. Then down and step back with both feet. Step forward leading with the opposite leg, therefore putting the other leg in the air. Pump your arms at the same time. Repeat for about 30 seconds.

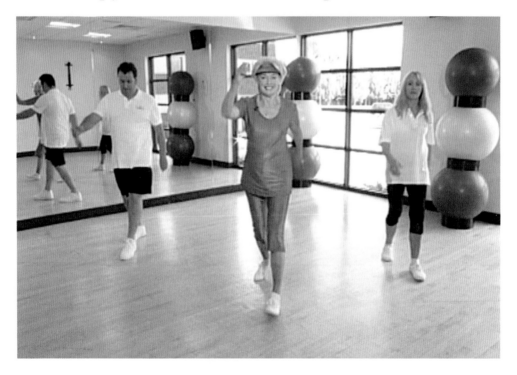

Marching on the spot for beats 1, 2, 3, 4, then squat down, hold for a few beats, then come up in time with the music and repeat this sequence for about 30 seconds.

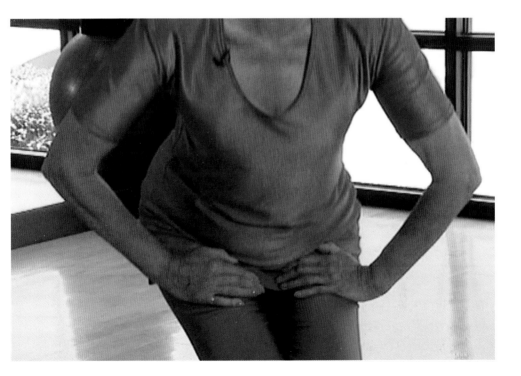

Move two steps sideways and clap, then two steps the other way and clap – in time with the music. Repeat for about 30 seconds.

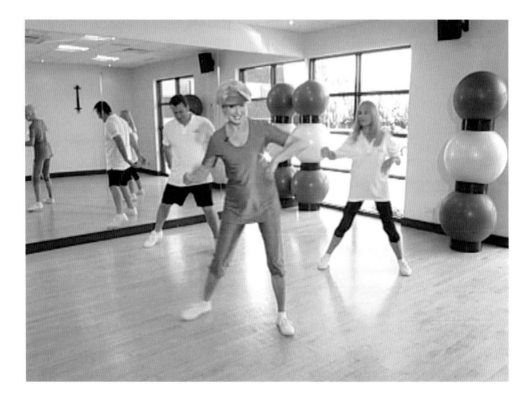

With quite a wide step, step from side to side swinging your arms up high as you take each step. The higher the arms go, the more aerobic the exercise. Continue the exercise for about 30 seconds.

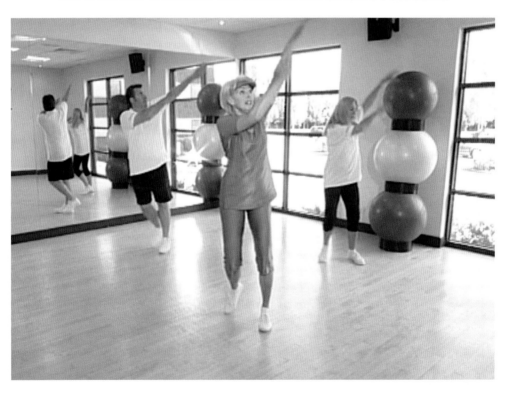

Chapter 3

Toning

Lie down with your feet on the floor.

For all toning exercises the correct posture must be kept at all times: a strong core must be engaged by making sure that there is no arch in your lower back, and by pulling in the tummy and pushing your waist to the floor with the pelvis tilted slightly forward. Always breathe in and breathe out during the exertion.

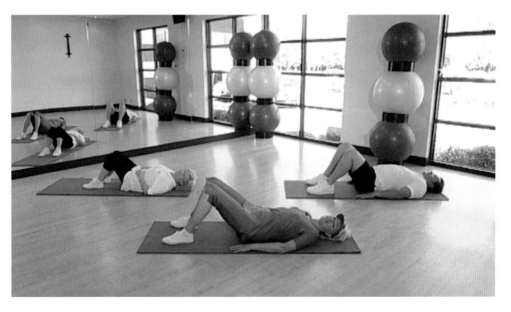

Put your hands on your thighs and push your hands towards your knees, lifting your head and shoulders off the floor working your abdominal muscles. Then release back down and repeat about 10 times.

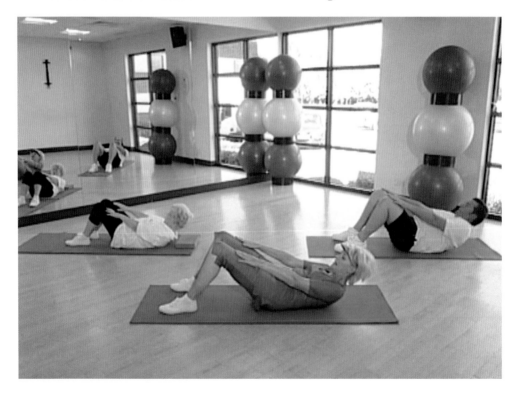

You can also put your hands to your head when doing the above exercise. Repeat about 10 times.

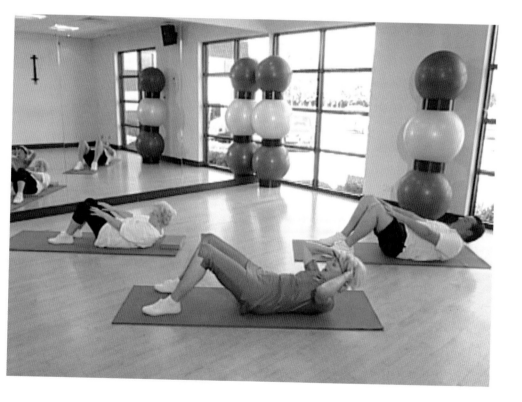

Take your right arm up and brush it past your ear and bring it back down to your side, then do the same with the left arm. Repeat this once more.

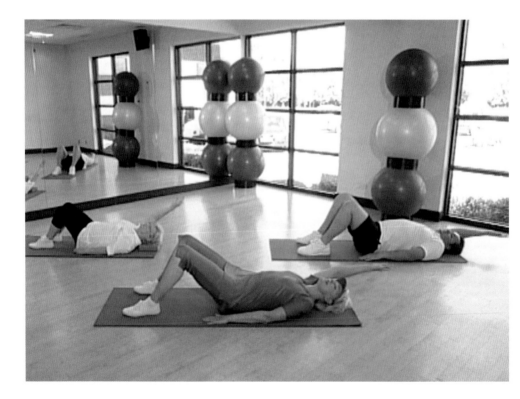

Take your right hand and lift across to the left knee – up and back. Do the same with the left hand. Repeat 4 more times.

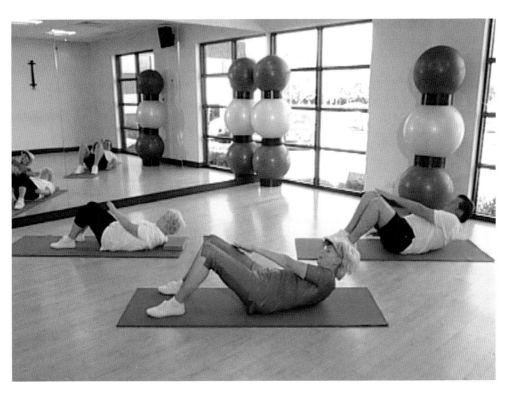

Put both arms down by the side making sure that your feet are firmly flat on the floor and then lift your bottom up – lift and then lower. Repeat 5 more times.

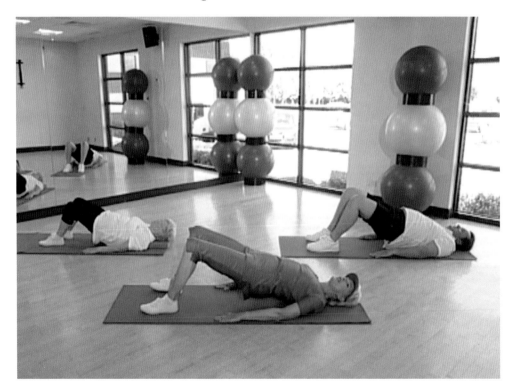

Push yourself up so that you're resting on your elbows. Keeping your tummy nice and taut then straighten out your right leg with your foot facing upwards. Lift the leg and then lower. Repeat 5 more times and then do the same with the left leg. Control the movement up and down at all times.

Step 1   Step 2

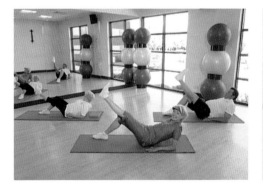
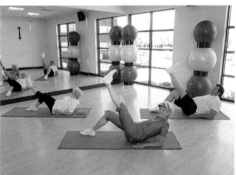

Sit up with your hands comfortably under your shoulders with your fingertips pointing towards your feet.

Step 1

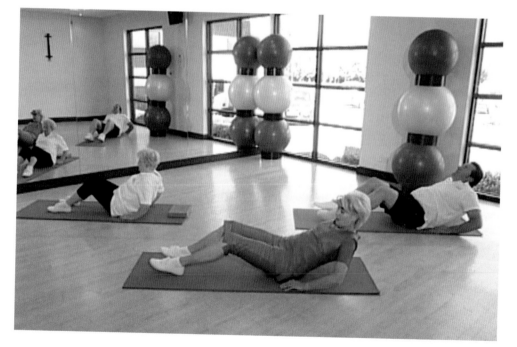

Relax down and then push back up. Repeat 5 more times.

Step 2

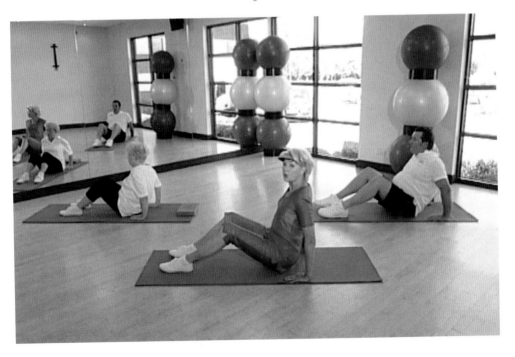

Lie on your side with the underneath arm totally outstretched or with your elbow propping your head up. Put the other hand in front of you and be careful not to roll forwards or backwards.

Step 1

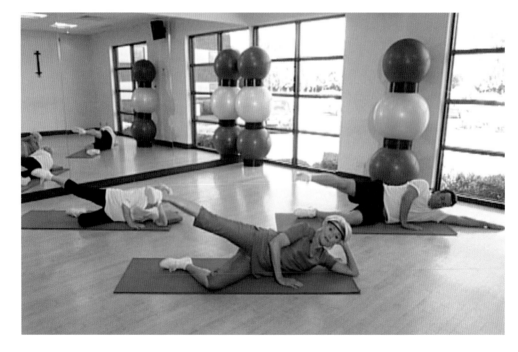

Bend both knees up, and then straighten the top leg with your foot crooked. Then lift that leg and then lower. Repeat 5 more times. Relax down and then push back up. Repeat 5 more times.

Step 2

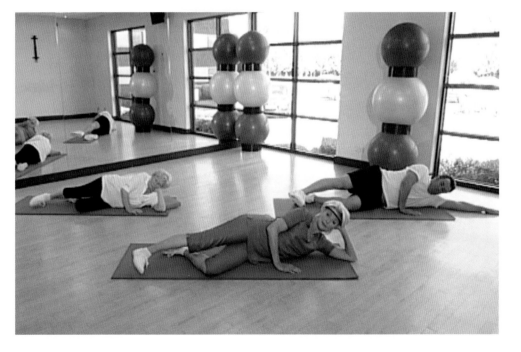

Bring the top leg down to sit on top of the lower one, straighten the lower leg and then let the top leg drop forward. Crook the foot on the lower leg and pulse the leg up and down for about 20 seconds.

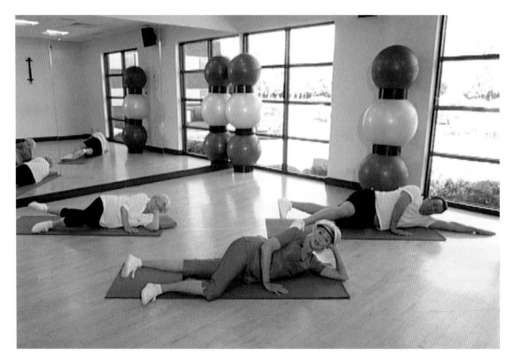

Roll over and repeat the last two exercises on the other side.

Lie on your tummy with your hands resting on your bottom and your head on the floor looking face down. Lift your head and shoulders at the same time – lift, and then lower. Repeat 8 times.

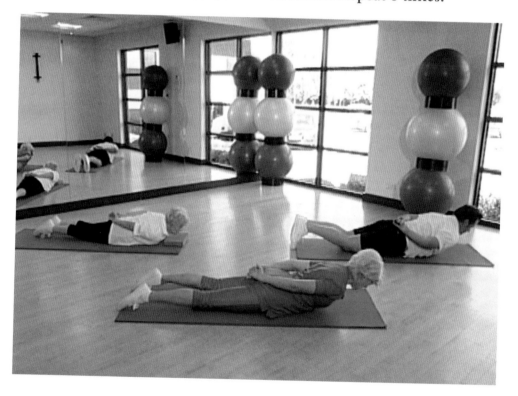

Come onto your hands and knees with your hands shoulder width apart. Straighten out one leg behind you with that foot crooked, then lift and lower. Pull up the tummy throughout and keep the head and shoulders in a straight line – do not look up. Repeat 10 times on one leg then do the exercise again on the other.

Step 1

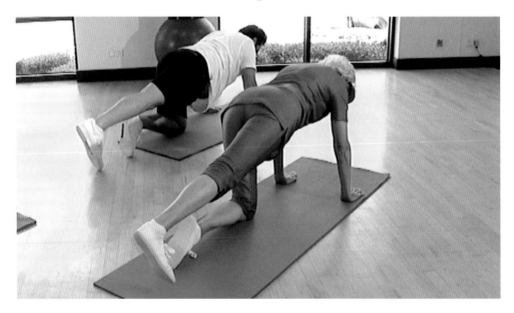

If you have a problem with your back you can do this with a half levered leg instead.

Step 2

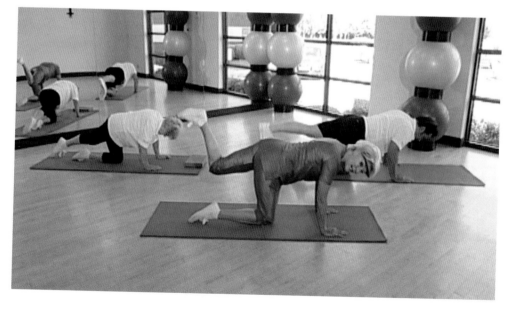

Sit on your mat with the right leg crossed over the left and with your hands comfortably to the side. Rock from side to side a few times.

Step 1

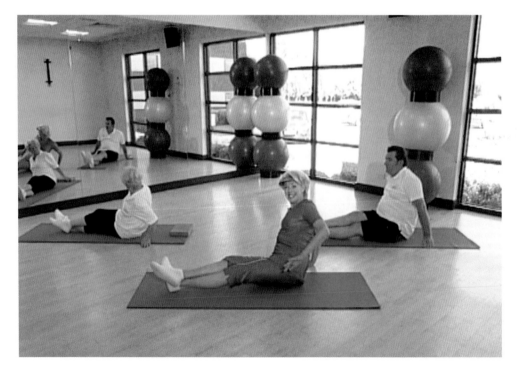

Put both hands out in front and continue rocking from side to side, pulling in the tummy at all times. Keep going for about 20 seconds.

Step 2

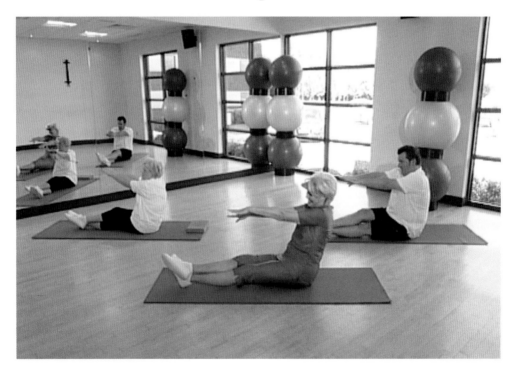

With your feet and hands straight out in front of you, move forward about a metre by bending your knees one at a time and wriggling your bottom.

Step 1

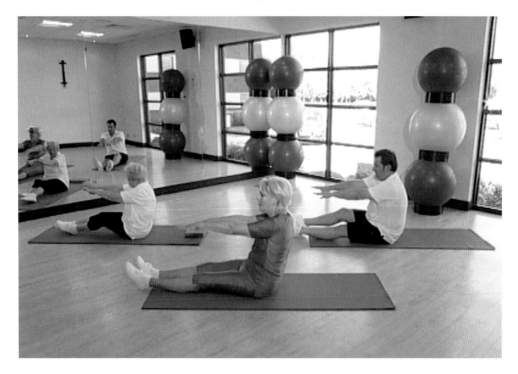

Put your hands down to the side and bring your feet up and then push through to move backwards again. Repeat.

Step 2

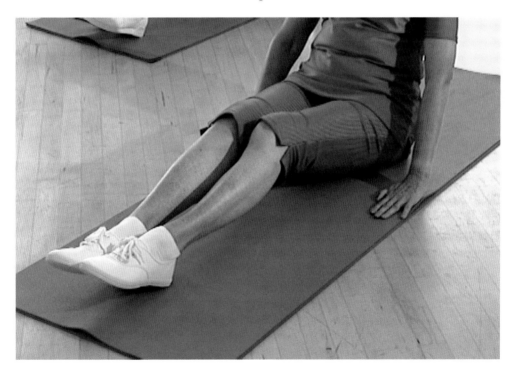

Chapter 4

Relax and Cool Down

For stretching the legs, lie on the mat with your knees bent and arms down by your side, with you're your tummy pulled in and your waist flat against the mat – no arched backs. Hug your right leg, point your toes and take it up so that it points at the ceiling with one hand behind your calf and one behind the thigh.

Step 1

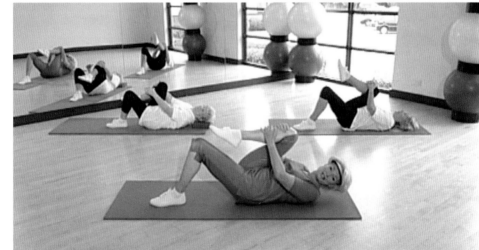

Hold for several seconds.

Step 2

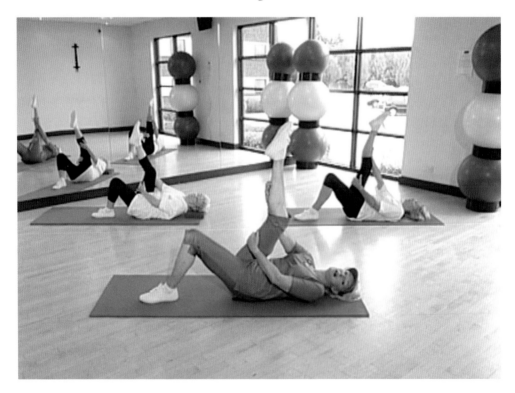

Then turn your toes towards you and you'll feel a different stretch. Hold.

Step 3

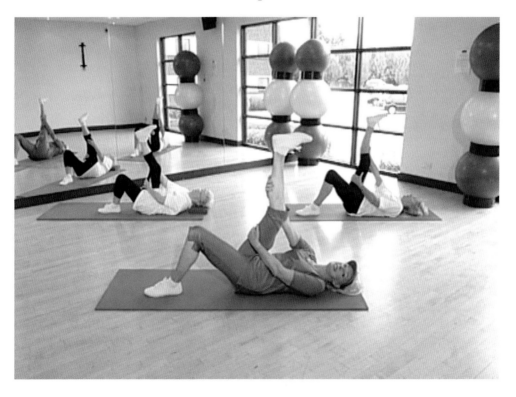

Take a deep breath and as you breath out pull the leg a little more towards you to increase the stretch – the leg doesn't have to be straight if you can't manage it. Hold for about 20 seconds.

Step 4

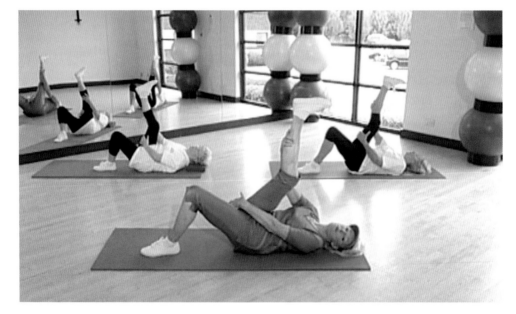

Repeat all of the above with the other leg.

For a lower back stretch, hug both knees in towards your chest and take your head to your knees, as far as is comfortable. Very gently rock from side to side.

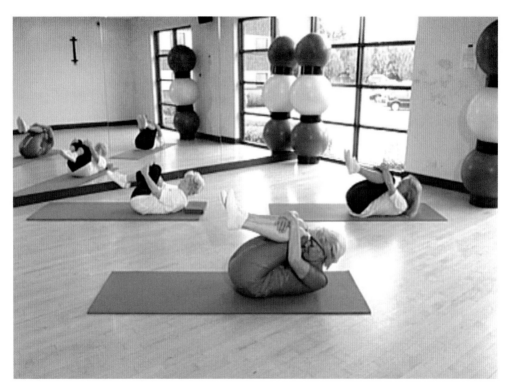

With your feet flat on the floor and close together, take your arms out to the side turning the palms of your hands upwards. Drop your knees over to the right and at the same time turn your head to look left. Only take your knees over as far as is comfortable for you. Hold for 20 seconds.

Step 1

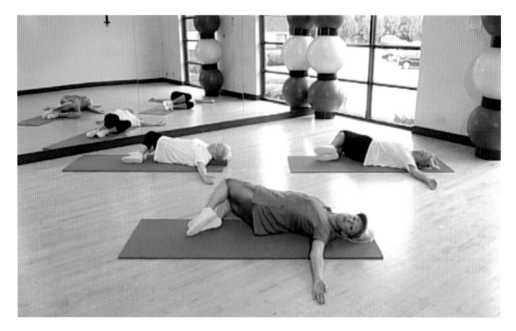

Slowly bring your knees and head back to centre and roll over to the other side. Hold for 20 seconds.

Step 2

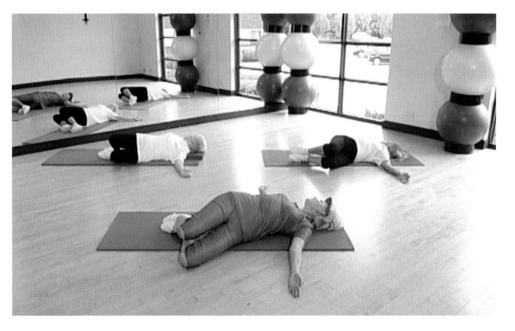

To stretch your quadriceps, lie on your left side with your lower arm supporting your head. Take your hand behind you, grab your ankle and either stretch away with the leg up or if you can, take the leg down keeping the front thighs parallel and bring the foot to your bottom. Hold for 20 seconds. Roll over onto your right hand side and repeat with the other leg.

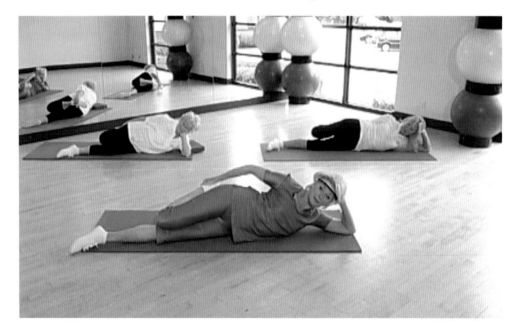

Roll over onto your tummy and place your arms with your elbows under your shoulders and palms facing down. Put your head on the floor and as you take a deep breath out push yourself up and stretch out through the abdominals. Hold for 20 seconds.

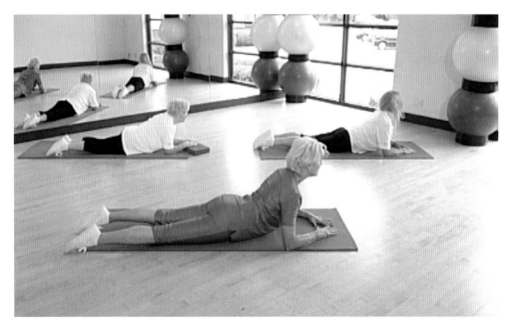

Move onto your hands and knees and walk your hands forward on the mat.

Step 1

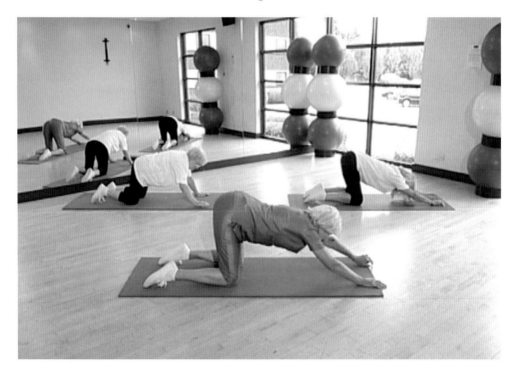

Stick your bottom out and drop your head down to the mat and feel a good stretch through your shoulders and back. Hold for 10 seconds.

Step 2

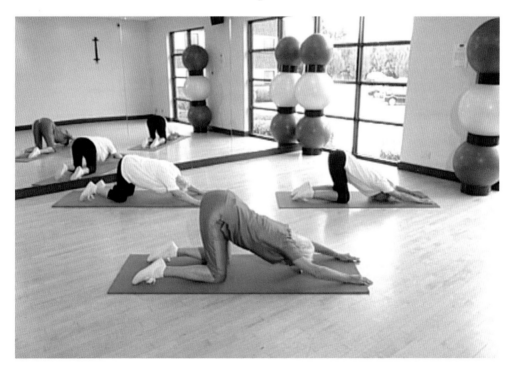

Come back up and then sit back onto your ankles and take both of your arms behind you, dropping your head down onto the mat. Hold for 20 seconds.

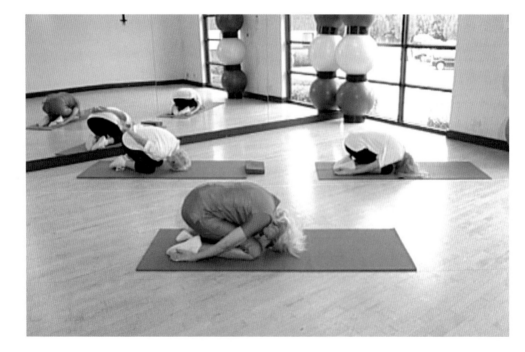

Move onto all fours with your hands underneath your shoulders and your knees shoulder width apart. Take a nice deep breath and pull up your tummy muscles, arch up your back, round out your shoulders and drop your head down so that you're looking between your legs. Hold for 20 seconds.

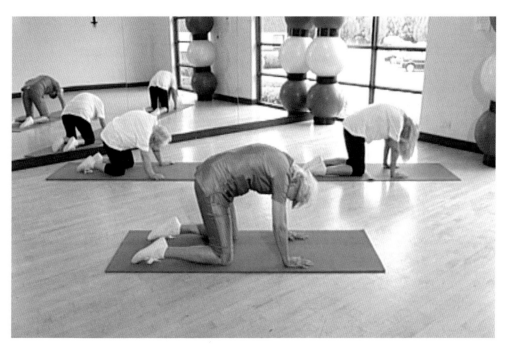

Relax the back down, stick your bottom out and lift your head up looking out. Hold for 20 seconds.

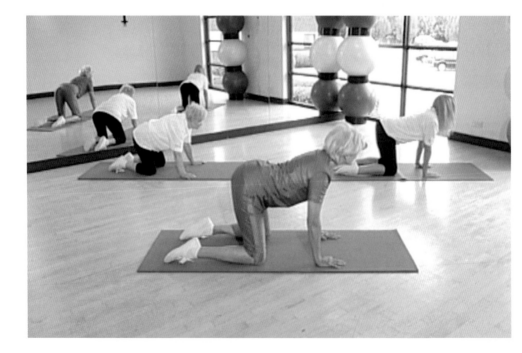

Sit with the soles of your feet together. Hold your ankles and pull your feet in towards you as much as is comfortable. Gently push down on your knees. Drop your head down to relax that at the same time and then gently roll the head from one side to the other – never roll your head back.

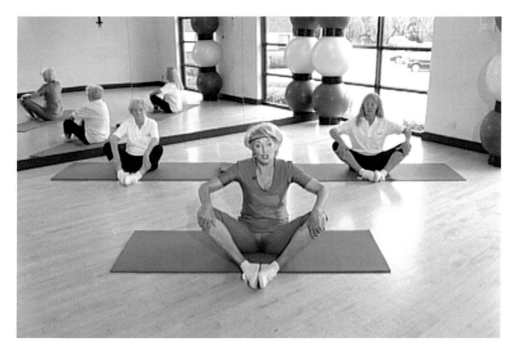

Lie on the mat with your knees bent, feet flat on the floor and hands down by your side. Lift the right leg, point your toes and let your leg slide away from you down the mat. Feel the stretch through the toes, ankle, knee and hip. Hold for 10 seconds and relax. Repeat with the left leg.

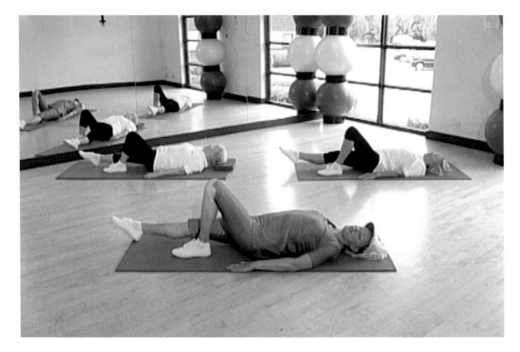

Lift your right hand up pointing your fingers towards the ceiling, stretching through the fingers, wrists, elbow and shoulder. Hold for 10 seconds.

Step 1

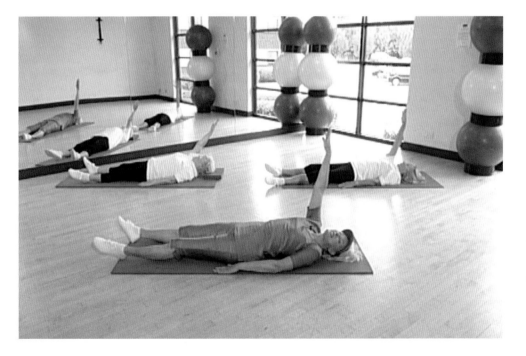

Then take the arm back over your head, just brushing past your ear.

Step 2

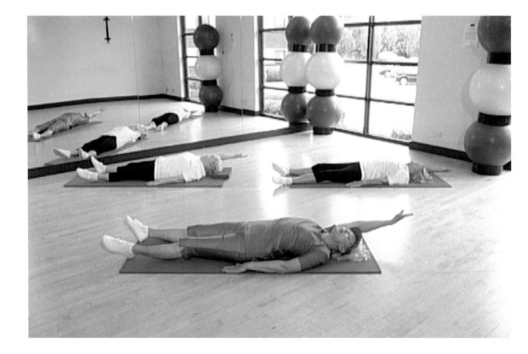

If this is uncomfortable, take the arm out to the side instead. Repeat with the left arm.

Step 3

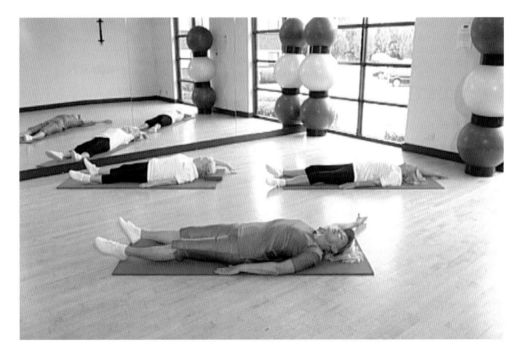

Move into a full body stretch, stretching through every possible joint you can. Hold for 10 seconds and then let your whole body relax.

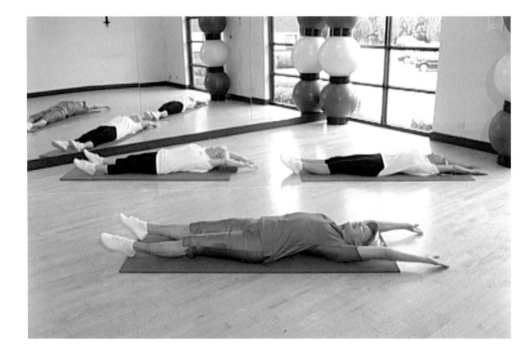

In a kneeling position with your hands on your hips take the right leg to the side, keep your foot facing forwards. Take the right arm into the air and take a deep breath. As you breathe out bend over to the left hand side. To extend the stretch put your other hand on the mat and hold. Come back to centre and repeat on the other side.

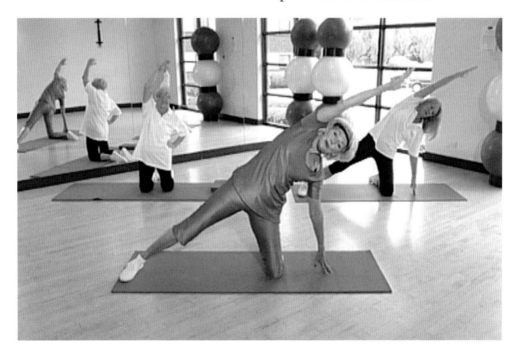

Stand up very slowly by uncurling the body with the head coming up last. Then stretch up to the ceiling and hold.

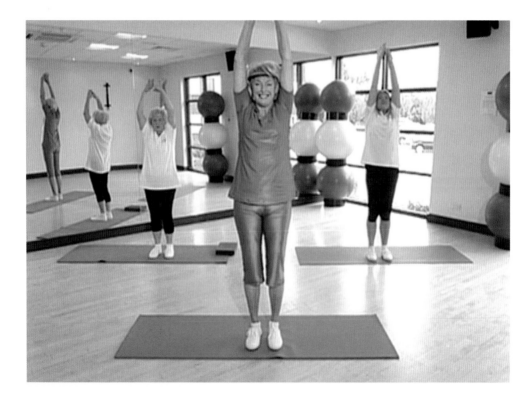

Chapter 5

Facial Exercises

All facial exercises should be performed sitting comfortably and right back on a chair with both feet on the floor (use some cushions if you need to to achieve this). Sit in front of a mirror.

The French Connection: say 'eh' to move your mouth back a little, then 'eeeee' to move it back further and finally 'ah' to open your mouth wide. Repeat twice more.

Step 1

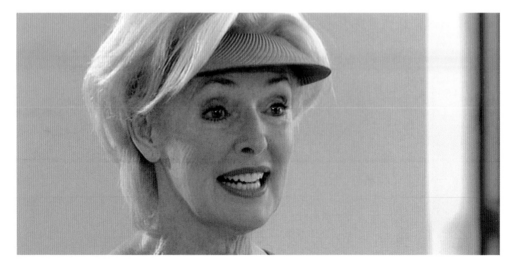

Step 2

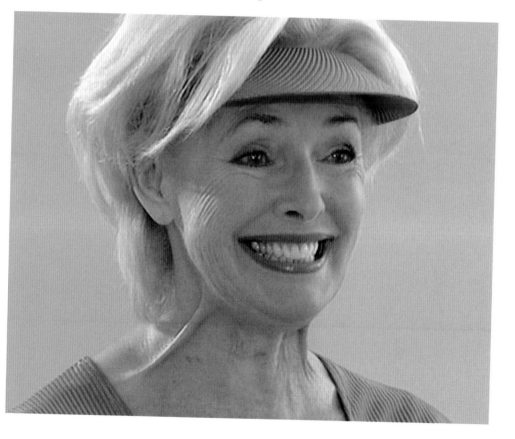

Step 3

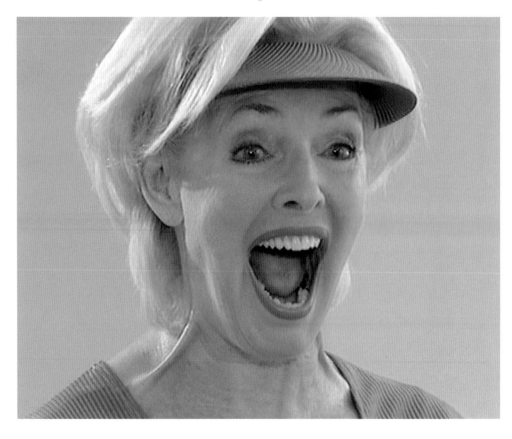

To retain a smiley face, make a tight lip across the teeth and then think about the corners of your mouth and your cheeks, and then lift and hold for a couple of seconds, then relax.

Step 1

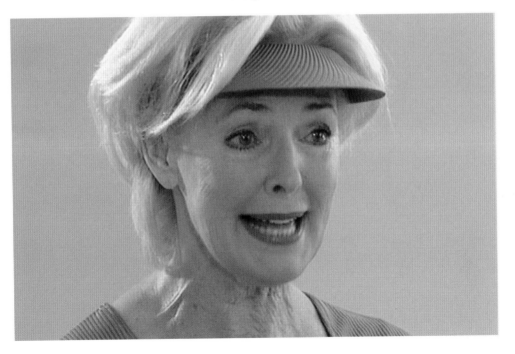

Repeat 5 times.

Step 2

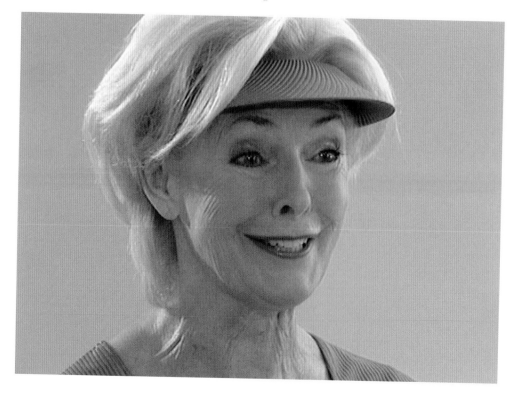

To work on your jowls, look in the mirror and just glug like a goldfish by opening and closing your mouth. To increase the effectiveness of the exercise lift your chin a little.

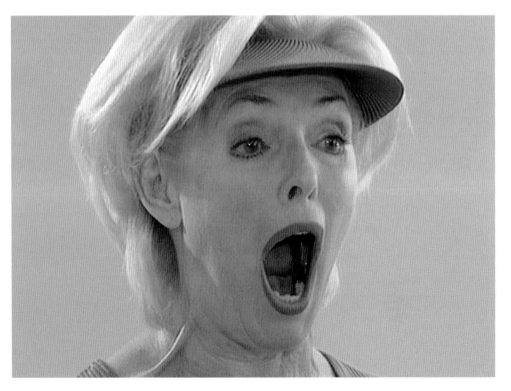

Another jowl exercise is called 'the Pelican'. Place your lower lip over your top lip and then move your head back to really feel the movement. Hold for a few seconds then relax. Repeat about 5 times.

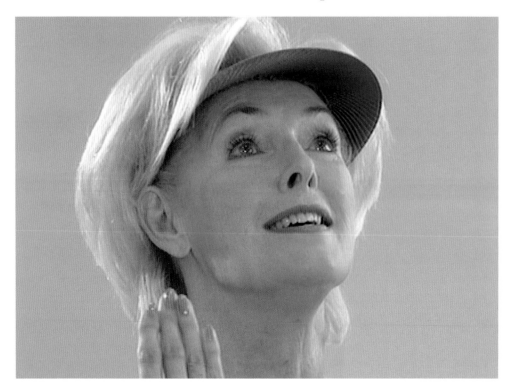

For baggy or droopy eyes do an exercise call 'the Uppers'. Put your index fingers softly under your eyebrows and close your eyes. When you open them you have to flicker, flicker, flicker, flicker your eyes by blinking as quickly as possible for about 10 seconds.

Step 1   Step 2

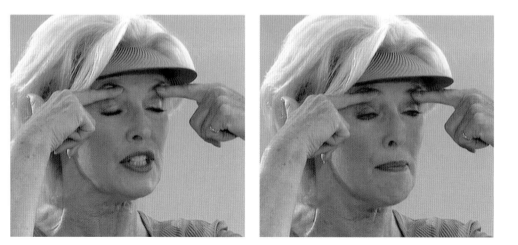

For nice bright eyes, sit looking at the mirror with your head straight.

Step 1

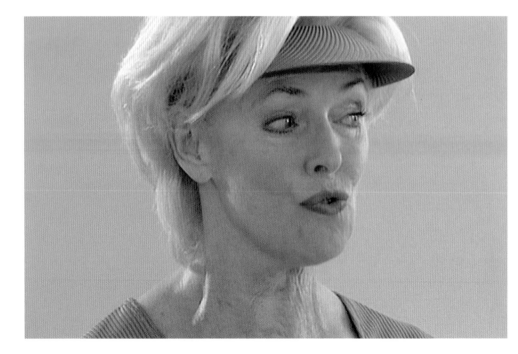

Take your eyes to the right then take the eyes up then to the left and then down, but don't move your head down, just move your eyes.

Step 2   Step 3

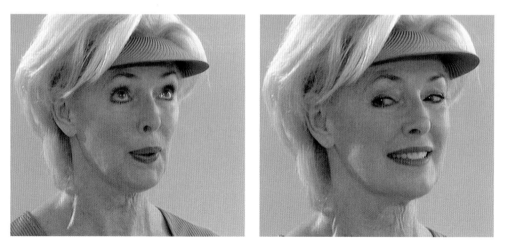

Repeat twice more, then blink and relax.

Step 4

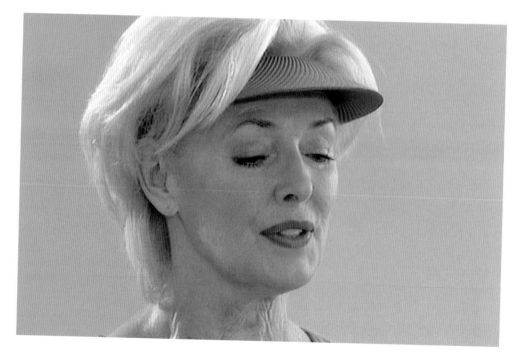

To feel energised, place your hands on your knees, close your eyes and count to three. Open your eyes as wide as you can, stick out your tongue to touch your chin if you can and at the same time spread your fingers and roar like a lion!

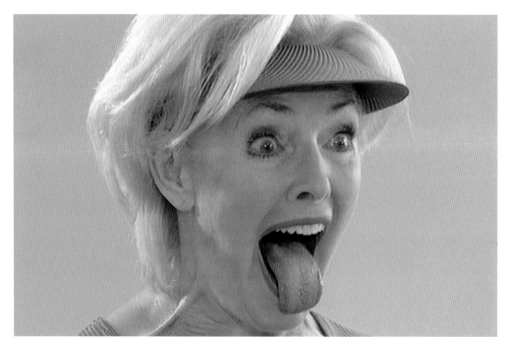

Design and artwork by Scott Giarnese

Published by Demand Media Limited

Publishers Jason Fenwick & Jules Gammond

Written by Michelle Brachet